LIVING YOUR BEST LIFE

BUILDING A BEAUTIFUL BODY AND SOUL

WILLI ASH

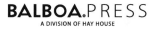
BALBOA.PRESS
A DIVISION OF HAY HOUSE

Balboa Press books may be ordered through booksellers or by contacting:

Balboa Press
A Division of Hay House
1663 Liberty Drive
Bloomington, IN 47403
www.balboapress.com
844-682-1282

Print information available on the last page.

ISBN: 979-8-7652-3893-6 (sc)
ISBN: 979-8-7652-3894-3 (e)

Balboa Press rev. date: 02/25/2023

Disclaimer

I wrote this book to share my experiences and the benefits I have received from using ESO: (essentials oils) in my healthcare journey, I'm not a license physician and this disclaimer is to make you aware that I'm not prescribing the use of ESO's. I'm just sharing my life experiences and the benefits I've had with using ESO's as a nurse whom has been dealing with chronic inflammation of my body, since my diagnoses Crohn's' disease at the age of 33.

Crohn's is an autoimmune disorder of the colon. I have been able to minimize episodes of G.I pain, diarrhea, fatigue and muscular weakness, by reducing my stress and anxiety with the use of essential oils. I also take a gut friendly probiotic daily. I encourage you to check with your physician prior to using any of the alternative measures written in this book, to make sure they're safe and will not interfere with your medications.

Contents

About the Author
Willi L. Ash B.A. EDU, L.P.N

I have been employed in the healthcare industry since 1979. I've enjoyed 44 years as a nurse and health and wellness educator. My career has and continues to be very rewarding.

Throughout my career I have worked and gained much knowledge from the many dedicated physicians, nurses and paraprofessionals, whom I admired and greatly respect.

I reside in Atlanta, Georgia.

The proud mother of three beautiful daughters Carisa, Kendra, and Stacia.

My compassion and dedication to the health and wellness of others led me to write this book in the hopes it will educate people how to thrive physically, mentally, emotionally and spiritually.

To live a healthy abundant life, which is what GOD'S wants for us all.

Chapter 1

Systems of the Body

Romans 12:1 I Beseech you therefore brethren, by the mercies of God, that you present your bodies a living sacrifice, holy acceptable unto god, which is your reasonable service.

1. *Integumentary System: The largest sensory organ that protects the entire body, which consist of the skin, hair, nails, glands, and nerves. The skins protect deeper tissues of the body as well as provides vitamin D syntheses, which means the skin is responsible for producing vitamin D during exposure to sunlight, the sun ultraviolet radiation penetrates into the epidermis (the first layer of our skin) and photolyzes provitamin 03. Therefore, the skin is the site for the synthesis of vitamin D and a target tissue for its active metabolite. The skin also regulates fluid and blood loss.*

2. *Skeletal system: Provides a frame structure for the body that consist of 206 bones, cartilages, and joints. Together these structures farm the human skeleton. The banes store calcium, protect our vital organs and produces red blood cells.*

3. *Muscular system: Consist of 700 muscles. Which are attached to the skeletal system. These muscles make up half of a person's body weight. Each of these muscles is a discrete organ constructed of the skeletal muscle tissue, blood vessels, tendons and nerves. Muscle tissue is also found inside the heart, digestive organs and blood vessels. The muscles provide energy to the body, generates heat, allows the body movement and helps retain our posture.*

4. *Immune System: Consists of a combination of many different systems that fight disease. The immune system also consists of a network of antibodies which include the, white blood cells, proteins, as well as the lymph nodes, the tonsils, thymus, bone marrow and the spleen.*

5. *Lymphatic System: A network of tissues and organs that primarily consist of lymph vessels, lymph nodes and lymph. The tonsils; adenoids; spleen; and thymus are all part of the lymphatic system. There are 600- 700 lymph nodes in the human body that filter the lymph before it returns to the circulatory system. The lymphatic system helps the body fight pathogens and maintain fluid balance, it also picks up fluids leaked from the capillaries, it supports the immune system and houses white blood cells.*

6. *Cardiovascular System: Consist of the heart, blood vessels and approximately 5 liters of blood, which is 1.2 to 1.5 gallons of blood circulating throughout our blood vessels and body*

7. *Urinary System: Consist of two kidneys, to ureters, and a urinary bladder and the urethra. The system removes waste from the blood and helps maintain water in the body along with fluid and PH balance and regulates the bodies electrolytes balance.*

8. *Digestive System: Consist of the mouth, throat, esophagus, stomach, small intestine, colon, rectum and anus. The digestive system breaks down food and delivers products to the blood for the nourishment of the body cells.*

9. *Endocrine System: Consist of the pituitary gland, thyroid, parathyroid glands, adrenal glands, pancreas, ovaries and testicles. The endocrine system is a collection of glands that secret hormones into the blood, which regulate growth development and homeostasis. Which is (the process to prevent and stop bleeding) It keeps the blood within a damage blood vessel. This is the first stage of wound healing. This involves coagulation of the blood that changes from a liquid to a gel. Intact blood vessels are central to moderating blood tendency to form clots.*

10. *Nervous System: Relays messages throughout the body nerve cells. The Nervous System consist of two main parts. The Central Nervous System and the Peripheral Nervous system. These include the brain, spinal cord, nerve fibers that branch off from the spinal cord and extend to all parts of the body, including the neck arms, torso, legs, skeletal muscles and internal organs.*

11. *Reproductive System: Creates offspring's. In the human reproductive system, the major organs including the external genitalia and many internal organs including gamete producing gonads. The external genitalia are the penis and vulva and the gamete producing gonads are the testicles and ovaries.*

12. *Respiratory System: Supplies blood with oxygen which allows it to deliver the oxygen throughout the body. The upper and lower respiratory tract consist of the nasal cavity, sinuses, pharynx, larynx, trachea, lungs, diaphragm and bronchi.*

I've given you a breakdown of each systems function and purpose as it relates to the importance of how wonderfully God designed each of us. It's up to us individually to cherish our bodies and our life, for it was given to us for a season and a price that we don't' and couldn't pay back even if we could. God wants each of us to have life abundantly with longevity and great health. Our bodies cannot function properly without each system. We are wonderfully and beautifully made in the image of God.

So it's time to learn how to live your best and abundant in your body.

The twelve systems of the bodies are groups of organs and tissues that work together to perform important functions for the body.

The health and wellness of our bodies is effected by many factors some through environment as well as our family genetics and heredity factors. There are also many other known and unknown factors, which may also contribute to chronic and acute illness that we a loved one or a friend maybe suffering with today.

Chapter 2

Category of Disease

Luke 4:23 Physician heal thyself

Is a true word of faith and believing what a man thinketh so is he? We have to daily speak life over ourselves to manifest a healed body.

So before we get into how disease affects our body, I want to discuss the category that diseases fall under. Which are communicable and non- communicable disease.

Communicable Diseases: Which are caused by pathogens and can be transferred from one person to another or from one organism to another in humans such as measles, food poisoning and malaria to name a few.

Non-communicable Diseases: Which are diseases that are not transferred through people or other organisms, such as Cancer, diabetes, heart disease, genetic disorders and neurological disorders as well as others factors that can have major effects on physical and mental factors

There are other factors that contribute to disease such as, alcohol. Smoking, stress, drugs, and daily situations that may occur in our lives.

The above listed categories also come under these 4 main types of disease.

- *Infectious disease - such as hepatitis B, hepatitis C, tuberculosis, malaria and dengue (a mosquito- borne occurring in tropical and sub- tropical areas). HIV, chicken pox, influenza, common cold and many others that are caused by bacteria, fungi, parasites, and viruses.*
- *Deficiency diseases - A disease caused by a lack of some essential important element in the diet, usually a particular vitamin or mineral, such as vitamin A, B1, B2 complex, vitamin C and other minerals needed to promote a healthy body and organ function. Such ae the lack of vitamin A - visual and skin changes, vitamin B12 can lead to anemia, Jack of vitamin C- Scurvy, lack of vitamin 0- Rickets and bone abnormalities, vitamin B2- growth retardation as well as bad skin, lack of vitamin E- can lead to neurological problems and the lack of minerals- in the body can lead to magnesium deficiency, goiter which is known as an enlarge thyroid. There are so many other illnesses and diseases that develop from*

lack of vitamins and minerals, but I'm unable to name them all, but I'm sure you get the ideal of how important they are to your body.

Hereditary diseases (including both genetic diseases and non-genetics hereditary diseases - Diseases that are passed down from parent to child such as, Downs Syndrome, cystic fibrosis, Hemophilia, Muscular dystrophy, Toy Sach and Sickle Cell as well as many other not mention. The heredity of our parents, grandparents as well as family genetic plays a part in how illness and diseases are transferred through DNA. you know the saying well my mother suffered with high blood pressure or my father suffered with diabetes so I inherited from my parent, so I just have to learn how to live with it. We can't control the transference of DNA, but we can control how and illness affects our body. Through lifestyle changes. Many times eliminating the use of medication, through exercise 3-4 times a week one of the best and most inexpensive exercises I know is walking and requires no gym membership or equipment, its stimulates the heart and lowers the blood pressure instantly with consistency, along with diet changes you can defeat any alignment

- *Physiological diseases- Consists of disorders such as, PTSD (post-traumatic stress disorder), eating disorders, anxiety, bipolar, depression, sleep disorders as well as neurological disorders.*
- *Death due to disease - Known as death by natural causes consist of diseases such as, cerebrovascular (aka Stroke and Ischemic heart disease) suicide, Diabetes, Cancer, Pneumonia, COPD (Chronic obstructive pulmonary disease), Alzheimer, Influenza kidney disease and un-intentional work related injuries. These are the most common related illness that lead to death in our society and effects both sexes. The most leading cause of death in men and woman today is heart disease. Remember it never too late make lifestyle changes in your life. The control to change no matter what you age is an individual choice. Control your destiny to abundant health and longevity.*

So, let's discuss, specific illness and some of the diseases that affect health and well-being.

Chapter 3

Inflammation How It Effects Your Body

Inflammation: is defined as a localized physical condition in which part of the body becomes reddened, swollen, hot, and often painful, especially as a reaction to injury or infection.

Chronic inflammation is a more serious inflammation that can leads to far more serious health situations, such as Lupus, arthritis, certain types of cancers, heart disease strokes or autoimmune disorders. Usually long term aliments several months to years.

Acute inflammation consists of redness, swelling and moderate pain. (ex. Bee sting) injury or infection. usually Short term aliments. Several days or less than a few weeks

Let's discuss how conditions grouped by organ and body systems impacts our bodies. Complementary and alternative and how these diseases impact multiple body systems.

The diseases commonly encountered include cardiovascular (heart) disease, cancer, stroke, chronic obstructive pulmonary(lung)disease, diabetes, arthritis, Alzheimer's disease, multiple sclerosis and Parkinson disease.

The above listed diseases are considered by many physicians and scientist worldwide to be the main diseases that affect the 12 systems of the body.

Of course there are many other diseases that are known under the category of acute and chronic diseases and illness that affect our bodies overall health and wellbeing, but they all fall under the categories of the above listed diseases.

Let's not forget that nearly all sickness, diseases, and illness of the body stems primarily from inflammation, destroy the source of inflammation and regain your health.

The way to begin is to start eliminating refined and processed foods, white flour and starches, sugar, dairy as well as wheat products.

Is it easy to do this NO its not I'm still a work in progress myself, but you can change any bad habit into a good one, if you tackle one area at a time and not become overwhelmed with how can I do this?

I've learned that if you focus on doing one change at a time for 21-30 days, such as saying to yourself I'm going to stop eating sugar and sugar products for 21 days, you will find yourself struggling at first, but by day 7-10 the sugar carvings will have subsided greatly for sugary sweets, cakes and pies etc., replacing sugary products with fruits and occasional dark chocolate, which is better for your health.

Do the same with refined white flours, for 21-30 days. Start with little steps get rid of all white process flours in your kitchen cabinets and consider purchasing almond flour, unrefined white organic flour, coconut flour, whole wheat flour as well as rice flour there are many brands. I personally like Cassava flour by(Pamela). Sprouts grocers carries it and a variety of different many other brands that are of good quality and you can find them reasonably priced. I've found Sprouts organic flours fruits and vegetables reasonably price and fresher. I've purchase many organic bulk items that I use often such as my herbs, essential oils, flours and miscellaneous items to be more cost effective /lower in prices. from Amazon.

Research U-Tube for information on how to use these flours in your recipes.

There's two books I'd like to recommend, which I myself have read and use by Dr. Blake Livingood titled Food Made Simple that has great recipes, I cook from it daily.

The second book titled Livin Good Daily by Dr. Blake Livingood he offers this book free, you only pay for shipping; it gives you a 21-day guide to experiencing real health.

The reason started my journey to better health and wellness, because I was sick and tired of feeling achy, frustrated, physically and emotionally drain every day.

So I started researching journals, websites, reading books on different herbs and plants that aid in the healing of the body. Listening and studying the use of Aromatherapy and how it relates to assisting in healing of illness and diseases which affect our health.

I made a commitment to educate myself by following the teaching of knowledgeable Drs. of Naturopathic medicine, so I could pay it forward to everyone that is seeking and desiring to obtain an abundant life and longevity.

My journey to living a healthier lifestyle started when my mother begins suffering with water retention in both her legs and around her heart in her early 60's. She was eventually diagnosed with congested heart disease, after a year or so of medical treatment with her physicians her body didn't show much improvement, she had to eventually go on dialysis three times a week, which meant she had to go on a machine that removed her blood into a cycling process that took up to 3-4 hours each session to remove poisonous toxins from her body, the process was grueling and left her very fatigued afterwards, because her kidneys had been destroyed from years of uncontrolled high blood pressure. It broke my heart to see my mother go thru this 3 times a week, so I decided at that moment to aid my mother with my nursing skills and begin researching alternatives methods through diet changes_. and alternative medicine to enhance her life. Although the damage to her kidneys was irreversible, I looked for methods to add years to her life.

I started with eliminating salt from her diet using salt substitutes like Ms. Dash, herbs to season her foods and lower her blood pressure limiting her water intake, because it caused fluid retention that she wasn't able to eliminate, due to lack of her kidney function. My sibling and I aided her to get out of the more took her on outings, which aided her mental stability. We encouraged gradual diet changes we more fruits and vegetables and less fatty oils and meats that clogged her arteries. My mother was reluctant to change, but seen the benefits in the long run, she started to fill better less tried and fatigued after her dialysis treatments. These changes gave her 14 added years to her life.

Chapter 4

The Culprits of Inflammation

I Corinthians 6: 19-20: Do you not know that your body is the temple where the Holy Spirit resides a gift that Jesus gave to each of us when he died on the cross for our sins. So that we would be able to make choices that would benefit not just our lives but our families too. You are not your own You were bought with a price. Therefore, honor God with your bodies.

How our body fights inflammation?

Inflammation as stated previously is the body's natural response to safeguard against foreign bacteria, virus, and infection. When it senses a threat, the body will trigger the release of chemicals and the white blood cells (our bodies germ fighters). Certain inflammatory conditions or autoimmune diseases such as rheumatoid or osteoarthritis, fibromyalgia, celiac disease, Crone's disease and multiple sclerosis, the immune system reaction is inflammatory, even when there is no threat. The result damages internal tissues, causes high blood pressure, painfully swollen and stiff joints, and encourages the growth of abnormal cell (i.e. cancer cells)

Foods to Avoid to Decrease Inflammation in The Body

Dairy: use milk alternatives such as Almond, rice, hemp or organic soy. I found soy milk to also be inflammatory to women it counteracts with the estrogen in our bodies that caused me to feel fatigued and achy in my joints through trail of elimination I discovered that I was allergic to Soy and soy products.

Red meat which is linked to Chronic diabetes, heart conditions and cancer lingers in our bodies researchers say up to twelve to fourteen days in our digestive systems, which can cause toxic build up to cause our bodies to become sluggish, decrease energy and a feeling of heaviness.

Cheese: Including cream cheese

Margarines and other spreads that are high in trans-fat or partially hydrogenated oils, instead use clarified butter like ghee, olive, coconut grapeseed and coconut oils.

Processed cured meats, fatty red meat, or those meats that are preserved with salt, nitrates, nitrite or sugars for longevity and flavoring, such as hotdogs, sausages bologna and other lunch meats) are known inflammatory offenders that have been linked to autoimmune conditions.

Alcohol in excess causes chronic inflammation. Especially to the liver can is also linked to heart attack, strokes, peripheral artery disease, vascular disease, dementia and cancerous tumor growth over time.

Vegetable oils a diet high in omega 6 fatty acids can cause inflammation. You can reduce inflammation by substituting omega 6 oils (i.e., soy, sunflower, and safflower) with an oil rich in omega 3's common sources of plant oils rich in heart healthy omega 3 fatty acids include extra virgin olive, expeller pressed canola oil flaxseed oil, hemp oil, walnuts soybeans and Tofu, which can easily be exchanged in most cooking recipes.

Food additives: Popular additives, such as monosodium glutamate (or MSG) and aspartame have been linked to aggravating inflammatory symptoms in those with existing conditions (i.e. chronic asthma).

Sugar: The American Journal of Clinical Nutrition reported that processed sugars are among some of the foods we consume that cause our bodies pain by increasing inflammation overheating, redness and swelling. Our immune system is flagged which triggers inflammation when our bodies consumes bacteria, a food allergy or encounters an imbalance like our blood glucose levels.

Refined Carbohydrates: We've been taught to stay far, far away from carbs, but in reality not ALL carbohydrates are bad. We have been eating unprocessed carbs like grasses, roots, and fruits for millions of years. What is true is that refined carbohydrates., which have a higher glycemic index than unprocessed carbs, cause inflammation in the body. Refined carbs have had most their fiber removed. Fiber promotes fullness, improves blood sugar controls and feed the beneficial bacteria in the gut. Basically they've been stripped of all their good. Good carbs: are plant foods, whole grains, beans, vegetables and fruits. On the other hand, bad carbs are sugars, and refined white grains like white bread and rice.

Tropical Fruits: Some fruits contain a higher amount of fructose than others, so they should be eaten in moderation, bananas, oranges, mangos. Papayas and pineapples are fruits that should be eaten once a week especially if you're a diabetic.

Trans Fat: We know trans fats are bad for us but did you know that trans fats are the cause of inflammation, by damaging the cells that line our blood vessels. some trans fats are unavoidable since they do sometimes occur naturally in certain foods. The majority are manmade, which is why it's hard for the body to process and results in inflammation. Read the labels on the package foods you buy particularly look for and avoid any foods made with hydrogenated and partially hydrogenated oils.

Refined Grains: Foods like pasta, pizza, cereal and white bread should not only be eaten in moderation but avoided as much as possible. This is because when refined grains are consumed, they quickly breakdown into sugar, which causes inflammation. A diet high in refined grains leads to a greater concentration of inflammation in the blood, while a diet high in whole grains results in lower concentration of inflammation. Remember white breads are among the worst inflammatory foods because it's been stripped of all its nutritional properties and left with only fast- digestion carbohydrates.

This goes directly against what our body needs.

Saturated Fats: Fats which have been found in animal fat have been found to cause inflammation in the body. Healthy gut bacteria changes after we consume saturated fats practically those dairy which is also present in many baked goods and processed foods this imbalance can trigger and result in inflammation and tissue damage.

Agave: Even though Agave is advertised as a healthier alternative. It is still loaded with sugar. Sugar suppress the activity of our white blood cells, which makes us more susceptible to infectious disease (cold, the flu and other illness) as well as cancer. Agave is 85% fructose, which is a type of sugar which can only be broken down by the liver cells as oppose to glucose which can be metabolized by every cell in the body Fructose in particular puts p strain on the liver causing the accumulation of liver cells called non- alcoholic fatty liver disease, which can cause functioning impairment of the liver.

Chapter 5

Leaky Gut Syndrome

Psalm 103:3 who forgiveth all thine iniquities and who healeth all thine diseases.

I've informed you about the systems of the body, the food groups and their importance to our livelihood and detoxification of your body to eliminate harmful bacteria, waste, prevention of infections, which aids the body healing process, which promotes a better functioning body.

In order to maintain optimal health and wellness of your body we first have to recognize and destroy the culprits which is the root cause of the symptoms. The majority of chronic illnesses, aliments, diseases, and acute sicknesses that attacks our bodies generates from Leaky Gut Disease Heal your gut and you can heal your body, you have to target the root cause in order to get rid of the symptoms.

Leaky gut syndrome is also referred to as increased intestinal permeability, think of the lining of your digestive tract like a net with extremely small holes in it that only allows specific substances to pass through. Your gut lining works as a barrier keeping out bigger particles that can damage your system.

When someone has leaky gut the net in your digestive tract get damaged, which causes even bigger holes to develop in your net, so things that can't normally pass through, are now able to. Some of the things that can now pass through include proteins like gluten, bad bacteria and undigested foods particles. Toxic waste can also leak inside your intestinal wall into your blood stream causing immune reaction.

Leaky Gut Progression- Stress, Toxins, food particles, Drugs, Pathogens, organ Malfunction

- *GI Inflammation*
- *Food intolerances*
- *Immune System Issues*
- *Autoimmunity*

Leaky gut symptoms and progression leads to inflammation throughout your system and can cause symptoms such as:

- *Bloating*
- *Food sensitivities*
- *Thyroid conditions*
- *Fatigue*
- *Joint pain*
- *Headaches*
- *Skin issues like rosacea and acne*
- *Digestive problems*
- *Weight gain*
- *Syndrome X - Is a cluster of conditions that increase the risk of heart disease, stroke and diabetes*
- *Metabolic syndrome includes high blood pressure, high blood sugar, excess body fat around the waist and abnormal cholesterol levels. The syndrome increases a person risk of heart attack and stroke*

What Causes Leaky Gut?

There are four main causes of leaky gut which include:

- *Poor diet - A diet that doesn't consist of the 4 basic food groups*

- *Chronic stress - It weakens the immune system and cripples your ability to fight off bad bacteria and viruses, which can lead to inflammation and leaky gut. To reduce stress try getting more sleep, meditating on scripture, exercise 3-5 days a week, schedule fun into your week, allow yourself to rest at least one day a week, take the time to relax and try hanging out with positive people.*

- *Toxin overload- We come into contact with over 80,000 chemicals and toxins every single year, but the worst offenders for causing leaky gut include antibiotics, pesticides, tap water, aspirin and NSAIDS. You should consider buying a high quality water filter to eliminate chlorine and fluoride and look to natural plant based herbs to reduce inflammation in your body.*

- *Bacterial imbalance - Bad bacteria actually creates toxins called exotoxin that damage healthy cells and can eat a hole into your intestinal wall.*

The most common components of food that can damage your intestinal lining are the proteins found in un-sprouted grains, sugars, GMO's and conventional dairy. The problem with unsprouted grain is that they contain large amounts of antinutrients or nutrient blockers called phytates and lectins. Lectins are sugar-binding proteins that act as a natural defense system for plants that protect them from outside invaders like mold and parasites.

This is good news for plants but bad news for your body. Your digestive lining is covered with sugar-containing cells that block help break down your food. Lectins gravitate toward this area and when they attach to your digestive lining it damages your gut and causes inflammation.

Lectins and Foods that Because Leaky Gut add scripture from duet

Lectins are found in many foods, not just grains and consumed in smaller amounts your body will do just fine, but foods that have large amounts of lectins are more problematic. Some of the lectins and foods that because leaky gut include wheat, rice, spelt and soy.

Sprouting and fermenting grains reduce phytates and lectins, making these foods easier to digest. GMO and hybridized foods tend to be the highest in lectins since they have been modified to fight off bugs.

Gluten containing grains will damage your intestinal lining and cause leaky gut syndrome. So while you working to heal leaky gut and cure autoimmune disease, stay away from all grains, especially ones that contain gluten like wheat. Once your gut is healthy, you can add in grains that have been fermented and sprouted to eat occasionally.

Conventional cow's milk is another food that can cause leaky gut. Al casein iS a component of dairy that will harm your gut. Also the pasteurization process will destroy vital enzymes, making sugar lactose, which is difficulty to digest. The best dairy products to buy are raw unpasteurized milk products, such as goats milk, almond milk, kefir and many others check out the u tube channel or your internet for the different forms of nut milk and raw dairy products.

Sugar is a substance that wreaks havoc on the digestive system. Sugar will feed the growth of yeast, candida and bad bacteria, which will further damage your gut.

Leaky Gut effects the overall functioning of our entire body, mind and spirit this goes for adults and children.

Chapter 6

Optimal health through detoxing

Psalms 51: 10 Create in me a clean heart, 0 God and renew a right spirit with in me

Detoxifying Your Body

Detox is defined as a process or period of time in which one abstains from or rids the body of toxins or unhealthy substance; detoxification basically detoxification means cleansing the blood. This is done by removing impurities from the blood in the liver where toxins are processed for elimination. The body also eliminates toxins through the kidneys, intestines, lungs, lymphatic system and skin. However, when these systems are compromised impurities aren't properly filtered and the body is adversely affected.

Psalm 30:2 Lord my God. I called to you for help and you healed me

To acquire a healthy body and mind we will need to seek God for instructions and direction. Detoxing your body once or twice a year will help eliminate bad bacteria that lives in our gut (digestive tract) and contributes to inflammation., illness, fatigue and other diseases that contributes to sickness in the body.

How Do You Start a Detox?

First thing you can do is eliminate alcohol, coffee, cigarettes, refined sugars and saturated fats, all of which act as toxins in the body and are obstacles in your healing process. Try to eliminate or minimize the use of chemical based household cleansers and personal health care products such as, cleansers, deodorants, toothpastes, shampoos and substitute natural alternatives, also try to eliminate stress in your life or the stress triggers, what is known as the adrenaline rush, (over activity of the adrenal glands), which releases toxins in the body.

Meditation, walking, yoga, water aerobics or any form of light to moderate exercise that you enjoy.

Exercise at least 3 times a week minimum it will help your body thrive and maintain optimal health and overall wellbeing. Be sure to check with your doctor before starting any exercise program.

Which Detox Program Is Right for You?

There are many detoxification programs and detox recipes, depending on your individual needs. A seven-day detox program is most used, because it usually takes the body seven days to cleanse the blood.

A two day fast of juices and liquids that are all natural or organic works best to cleanse the blood and prepare your body for detoxing, but also make sure you drink plenty of water to flush out toxins, water intake is different for everyone examples) if you weigh 100 pounds your intake would be 67 ounces, if you weigh 240 pounds your intake would be 161 ounces you take how much you weigh and multiply it by 2/3 or 67 percent to determine what your water intake should be, prior to taking on the task of detoxing make sure you prepare yourself mentally as well as physically, because this is a major undertaking you're getting ready to prepare your body, it will go through withdrawals, possibly aches and pains as your body gets rids of toxic waste that has been trapped in your muscles, tissues, blood stream and organs, the first 2-3 days will be the hardest. Start slowly, by trying a 2-day detox and see how you feel then a 3 day until you are gradually able to do 5 to 7 days. We should try and detox are bodies at least 3-4 times a year or each time the seasons change. I found when I'm doing a detox cleanse I won't exercise, but meditate instead to help keep me focus on my goal. Strenuous exercise of any kind can cause too much pressure on your organs and body.

Remember no refined sugar juices or liquids which contain (fructose and refined sugars products) this will defeat the purpose of preparing your body for detoxing. Try and use all natural organic juices

Bone broth is a great liquid to drink during your detoxing it provides protein, calcium, phosphorous and potassium, you can buy organic bone broth in health food stores or online suppliers like Amazon, Swanson and locally through sprouts and whole foods.

To make bone broth yourself, you can use the bones of your favorite meat, such as, chicken, ham, turkey, oxtails and beef bones. Put bones in a large pot and fill with filtered water and simmer on low for 20 hours. You may add one chopped carrot, two stalks of celery chopped and your favorite herbs such as rosemary, thymes parsley or oregano to flavor your stock. Let cool and strain drink a cup daily or you may freezer broth in freezer bags and use in cooking your favorite dishes or recipes instead of water. Check out Shape.com for healthy eating and healthy cooking recipes with bone broth.

How Do You Know If You Need to Detox?

- *Unexplained fatigue*
- *Sluggish elimination*
- *Irritated skin*
- *Allergies*
- *Low grade infection*
- *Puffy eyes or bags under the eyes*
- *Mental confusion*
- *Bloating*
- *Menstrual pain*
- *Thyroid condition*
- *Joint pain*
- *Headaches*
- *Weight gain*
- *Digestive problems*

Today we live in a very toxic environment and these symptoms can also be associated with medical conditions. Be sure to consult your healthcare provider if you have questions whether detoxing is right for you.

Upon completion of your detoxing introduce solid foods back into your regimen slowly the first day consume light soups and broth if you handle that well introduced some light solids vegetables and fruits and gradually add meat, you don't want your body to go into a shut down or develop pain in your digestive system which could happen and cause your experience to be non-rewarding, to you mentally, you may even decide detoxing is not for me.

Believe me it's very beneficial when it done the right way you will fill a lightness in your body an overall wellness your taste buds for foods will change become sharper. A lot of foods you craved to eat prior to detoxing will diminish your craving, your food choices will become healthier because you will have a desire to continue to feel great and not allow all your sacrifice and hard work to go to waste. The only way that happens if you go back to eating your old way.

Remember anything worth having is worth scarifying for, so if you want abundant health decreasing /eliminating illness and diseases put you first. Say to yourself every day.

It's ok to put myself first.

I'm a priority.

My health is important to me and I will make it a priority.

My life is what I make of it.

I'm in charge of my success.

I can do all things through Christ who strengthens me.

For the days when you feel like giving up remember just how precious you are to God, yourself and your family.

Chapter 7

Detox Diets

Proverbs 3: 5 Trust in the Lord with all thine heart, and lean not unto thine own understanding. It's important to seek God's help before starting or choosing a detox regimen.

Five Favorite Detox Diets:

- *Simple Fruit and Veggie detox- the fruit flush detox, you eat lots of fruits and vegetables raw and cooked for five days you may also drink bone broth to maintain protein and cook your vegetables to add needed protein and nutrients for your body.*

- *Smoothie Cleanse - A mixture of fruits vegetables and herbs blended together and consumed 4-6 times throughout the day when hungry. Nutri Bullet is a good appliance for making smoothies or a blender.*

- *Juice Cleanse - Also known as juice fasting is consuming only fruits and vegetables, while abstaining from solid food for two to seven days, be sure add bone broth or protein powder for added nutrients.*

- *Sugar Detox- A sugar detox consists of eliminating sugar from your diet and cleansing the body. The best way to do this is cold turkey. Sugar detox cleanses the body and mind of especially depression, brain fog, fatigue as well as forgetfulness, easy to do NO! but very beneficial. Drink plenty of water to flush toxins from the body.*

- *Hypoallergenic Detox - Is also known as the elimination diet. removing foods from your diet that you suspect your body can't tolerate. This detox is used for people whom have a very sensitive gut or food allergies.*

- *Intermittent fasting - Setting a start and stop time for eating. (such as) begin your first meal at 11om and end your last meal at 7 not later than Bpm everyday allowing your body to burn fat as you rest this would take some discipline and meditation on your part, but it can be done, I've tried it, remember to drinking water throughout the day to help the body eliminate waste and toxins, this detox also can aid in weight loss and assist you in developing a healthier eating pattern.*

I reiterate make sure to drink plenty of water per day to increase the removal of toxins from the body. It is not recommended to detox any longer than three to seven days for safety and prevention of vital nutrients, minerals and vitamins that are necessary for proper functioning of your body. These detoxes can be done longer with the supervision of a doctor or certified naturopathic holistic professional. Be sure to inform your medical doctor of your desire to detox, also do not stop any prescribes medications without your doctors permission.

Chapter 8

Nutrition

1 Corinthians 10:31 - So whatever you eat or drink or whatever you do, do it all for the glory of GOD The four basic food groups consist of the meat, fruit, vegetable, milk and the bread group.

- *There's also another group that's not mentioned in the four basic food groups, but it is essential in the functioning of our bodies. This group is called the healthy fat and sugar group. Our bodies need healthy fats and sugar, which fuels our bodies and provides energy. The fat and sugar group. So let's discuss the importance of the four basic food groups and the healthy fats and sugars and how the twelve systems of the body are supported by them.*

- *Meat group: Contributes protein, minerals, vitamins and fat and these nutrients are important for their beneficial effects on our wellbeing. Meat aids the Muscular system because it supplies needed nourishment to the blood vessels and cells of the Cardiovascular system, the Digestive system helps to break down and deliver the meat eaten and supplies the body with minerals, vitamins and fat to the blood for the body cells. However, some components of meats, such as saturated fats, can concur negative health consequences, such Atherosclerosis a condition in which plaque deposits form on the walls of the arteries and can lead to heart disease. It's up to you to weigh the pros and cons when you're choosing whether to include meat in your diet.*

- *Milk group: Provides nutrients that are vital for health and maintenance of your body. These nutrients include Calcium, Potassium, Vitamin D and protein. The health benefits of the milk group aid the skeletal system by improving bone strength, the integumentary system (the skin) by improving its texture and outer smoothness, and provides a stronger immune system, and a stronger immune system.*

- *Fruit and Vegetable group: Provides Low calories and high fiber as well as water, Low in fat, most fruit and vegetable are plant based and a healthy source of vitamins and minerals. They provide nutrients to the functioning of all 12 systems of our body by reducing cholesterol, boosting the immune system, decreases the risk of diabetes, heart disease and stroke, they provide a high source of antioxidants, which helps protect against cancer, boost skin health and wound healing. I consider the fruit and vegetable group to be the building block to the other three groups.*

- *Bread and Cereal Group: This group consist foods that are made from pasta, wheat, oats, corn, meat barley, this group is better known as the cereal grain group, which consist of grain breads, pasta, breakfast cereal, grits and tortillas these are also examples of grain.*

We need to be careful when consuming grains such as pasta, rice, breads, white flour because they turn into sugar, which can lead to unwanted weight gain and obesity, these grains should be eaten in moderation.

This group also aids the Digestive system with fiber, which allows our colon to eliminate waste normally. We should consume at least 6 serving of bread and grains per day, which aids in the relief of constipation and diarrhea, fiber also reduces the possibility of the formation of harmful toxins in the large intestines, by reducing the intestinal transit time of the food content. It also reduces the absorption of cholesterol in the large intestine, which require nitrogen for growth, which reduces the chances of cancerous changes in the cells by reducing the amount of ammonia in the large bowels.

The Skeletal System is supported by the bread and grain group, because it supplies minerals, vitamins and nutrients throughout the bodies joints, cartilages and bones. Fiber helps to form the skeletal system.

The Reproductive System is supported by the bread and grain group, it allows expected mothers through their placenta to nourish their unborn child through the fetus umbilicus the needed nutrients, vitamins, and fiber for its healthy growth and development.

- *The forgotten group (The Fats and Sugar): Fats, Oils and Sugars do not fall under the actual food group, so they are put in the other category. Some oils in a diet are necessary to stay healthy. A few examples of these oils are vegetable oils such as canola oil, olive oil, soybean oil, corn oil and foods naturally high in oils, such as nuts, olives, some fish such as, salmon and avocados. Some foods we eat and drink don't fit into this group, examples are foods that contain extra fats, such as butter, margarines, sauces and salad dressings. Other examples are foods and drinks that contained extra sugars such as syrup, honey, jelly, jams, sugar, candy, fruit drinks, fruit punch, and sweetened soft drinks. These foods and drinks give us calories but few or no vitamins and minerals.*

These are extras to be consumed in small amounts once you get the foods you need from the food groups. Consuming foods or drink with extra fat and sugar will cause you to consume too many calories and not enough vitamins and minerals your body needs.

Many foods that contain extra fats and sugars come in light, fat free, low calorie or no calories, varieties such as light or fat free salad dressings and low calorie or no calorie sports drinks and soft drinks. These versions are a lot lower in extra fats and sugars -or may have none at all, so they're usually a lot lower in calories too. They are usually made with artificial sweeteners, such as fructose corn syrup, sweet and low, Splenda, equal These products should also be consumed in these in moderation, because they are not considered healthy sugars or fats.

- *Healthy fats Examples: Plant base oils are the best oils to use, such as are Corn oil, sunflower oil, safflower oil, canola oil, soybean oil which contains omega 6 a polyunsaturated fat that may help reduce insulin resistance and inflammation. Plant base vegetable oil typically mixes two types of fats, which are polyunsaturated and monounsaturated. When possible cook with Olive oil rather than butter, stick margarine or lard. Eliminate trans fats from your diet hydrogenated or partially hydrogenated vegetable oils even if it claims to be trans1at free.*
- *Saturated fats: Primary source includes: red meat, butter, lamb, pork, lard, chicken skin, cheese, ice cream, lard, tropical oils such as, coconut oil, palm oil. Use when possible Organic coconut oil grapeseed oil and olive oil. Also when buying cheese and ice cream try buying nondairy cheeses and ice cream, remove the skin from your chicken prior to cooking it. Try to eliminate red meat, Jamb, pork from your diet. When possible.*

If you must eat red meat, pork and lamb purchase grass fed meats when possible.

If possible it's also a good idea to buy food in bulk (large quantities) when possible and on sale for later use for your families, depending on the size of your family vacuum sealing your produce, fruits and meats is best to prevent excessive air and preserves your foods nutrients along with providing longer storage life, by as much as 6- 12 months. A good investment, since there many brands available today that are affordable (such as) The Seal a Meal or a product of that type, you'll be able to store fruits, vegetables, meats and some grain products without the worry of freezer burn also make sure you to label and date items before freezing.

Nutrition is the building blocks to a healthy body mind and spirit and I learned through taking care of mother that I needed to started nutritional changes in my own life, after reading many articles and journals on nutrition. I gradually decided what would be the easiest thing I could eliminate first, so I started with unhealthy fats as listed above and gradually introduced healthy fats and oils into my daily eating and cooking regiment, for 21 - 30 days and at the end of the 30 days I had developed a routine and found out theses oils made my food taste better and reduced my cholesterol and plaque buildup in my arteries.

My next challenge was the bread and cereal group, because I love bread, pasta, rice, cereals, and starches of all kinds. I found alternative flours that I could use in my baking that were healthier. My favorites are coconut flour, almond flour and Cassava flour I found I can use these in any recipe that require white process flour. After using these flours for 30 days I never looked back at using any type of processed grains, or flours,

I started my next challenge, which was the hardest for me because of my love for sugar, took me longer than 30 days to transitions. I'm currently a work in progress. I discovered through researching why so many people as well as myself have a desire or carvings for sugar products such as, chocolate, cakes, pies and sugary products it's mainly, because it ignites are brain and releases dopamine, which is a neurotransmitter, which causes us to have addictive behavior a pleasurable high from eating sugary products, so I found out the only way to eliminate sugar from my life was to go cold turkey and do a sugar detox, I know it sounds extreme but it's the only way to overcome sugar carvings, there's no easy

Way around it as your body goes through withdraws, replace fruit and 79% pure coco chocolate as a substitute it will make the transition easier on your mind and body, because sugar believe it or not is just as addictive as cocaine. I'm able now to resist sugar without feeling deprived. Fruits and vegetables were an easy transformation for me because I enjoy all types of fruits and vegetable. what I did learn was to buy them organic when possible. Buy quantity when in season and freeze them for later uses. You can store them up to 6 months to a year for later uses. If you can invest in a seal a meal sealer, it really preserves the freshness and flavor of your fruits and vegetables.

Milk products was also another hard challenge for me because I really enjoy ice cream (butter pecan) is my favorite and cheeses of all types. I could eat cheese everyday but I don't. I've limited myself to 2-3 times a week and when I do eat cheese I buy organic. My favorite ice cream is the so coconut brand. The changes that I had to get use to was the decrease in sugar the products had, but no lack in taste.

As far as milk products (Almond Breeze) is my favorite brand to drink. I even cook with it. Organic milk products are also good, just make sure it's not pasteurized and a brand you trust.

For every 21-30 days I was changing my eating lifestyle. I realize my desire for meat had lessen in my diet. I basically didn't have a desire for it anymore, but I added bake fish and chicken into my eating regimen, because I know I needed a source of protein other than Legume, which is beans. So I only ate those two meats when the desire for meat occurred. I eliminated pork, beef and other animal proteins.

Once I stopped eating those meats, when I tried to consume or re-enter them into my life, the taste was different, even when I purchase organic. Remember what the word says about eating clean and unclean meats. God stated that clean meats are fish with scales such as, salmon, grouper, snapper, trout and tuna. Many other such as catfish, shrimp, lobster, crabs and many other fishes of the sea are considered scavengers and don't have fins or tails. They are toxic to our bodies. Chickens, ducks, turkeys, geese, quail and pheasant are ok to eat.

Unclean meats as it states in Deuteronomy 1411-18 specifies that all clean birds can be eaten, but not the eagles, falcons, ravens, vultures, buzzards, seagulls, hawks, jackdaws (part of the craw family) storks and herons can be consume they are toxic to our bodies.

Most insects are not good to eat either, but some can be consumed, such as the locust, grasshopper and cricket theses are fine to consume.

God wants us to be holy for he is holy and treat our bodies as the temple where he dwells. Treat our bodies as a gift. Oh believe me I fall short in doing the things I know are against my health. We all do but we fall down, but we don't stay there we get up dusk ourselves off and keep trying till we get it right, because his mercy endures forever.

Chapter 9

Benefits of Essential Oils and Herbs

I remember as a child about the age of 8 years old, every winter one a week my grandmother would have my sibling and myself to come into the kitchen and line up behind each other in the kitchen to take cod liver oil what she called medicine to keep us healthy and protected from cold and flu bacteria that could cause us to get sick, boy did we hate that dreaded Cod liver oil regiment with a peppermint tea chaser to kill the oily test in our mouths, but it didn't help nothing curbed that fishy tasting oil it was horrible and we would all be gagging, before it was our turn to take I would bribe each of my sibling to go before me, so I could be last, thinking my grandmother wouldn't have any oil left in the bottle when it was my turn, oh well no such luck. She would let us know if it doesn't stay down you'll have to get another dose, my brothers could never keep it down and had to take another tablespoon The memory of how we acted causes me to laugh out loud.

Through my research I discovered that many ESO (essential oils) can be used for the same or similar conditions and illnesses, ESO such as Lavender and German -chamomile oil both are used for relaxation, but comes from different plants the variety offers you an option to find the oil that works best for you.

How does that saying go what works for me may not work for you?

I was amazed that(ESO) Essentials Oils are referenced in the bible over 600 times herbs over 68 times and get this frankincense, myrrh and galbanum essential oils are mentioned 54 times and were used the most by the physicians in biblical times because of their potency and multiple healing properties.

Essential Oils are and can be very beneficial in helping us maintain optimal health and wellness in our healthcare.

I will be discussing how ESO's can aid in healing the body of various illness and diseases and as well as the short and long term benefits of alternative naturopathic therapy.

There are more than 5-10 thousand illnesses as well as diseases in the United States that currently have no cure.

Chapter 10

The Integumentary System

Skin and Essential Oils

There are so many diseases, illness along with bacteria, fugues and viruses that effect the skin. You already know the skin is the largest system of the body that provides protection for the entire body, as well as our organs.

I learned the benefits of using essential oils, such as coconut oil, olive oil, almond oil grapeseed oil jojoba oil and avocado oil, these are essential and effective in uses for the skin and other regimen.

All of these oils and many others are very beneficial for beauty regiments, cooking, illnesses and diseases that may affect your health. The above listed oils are non- saturated oils, which are great for a healthy heart and blood flow.

Essentials(ESO) oil are good and effective, but remember to check with your physician and continue your prescribed medications if you have any skin conditions, such as Eczema, Atopic Der organic distributors. Doterra, Young Living, Planet Therapy, Now, Aura Cacia, but my favorites are Doterra and Plant Therapy.

The below listed oils are good for relieving skin disorders. Remember to use a carrier oil with any ESO's such as almond oil, coconut or whichever oil you find that works best for you, just remember the lighter the oil the easier it absorbs into the skin and your blood stream. Do not apply ESO's directly to your skin without adding it to a carrier oil, because it could cause severe skin rash and irritation.

- Peppermint oil -It's a universal oil that has cooling properties, which can help reduce itching caused by skin disorders and minor skin aliment such as poison Ivy, bug bites, it also calms itching that is related to diabetes, liver and kidney disease, which may cause some people extreme dryness of the skin, moisture loss and itching. This oil is great for alleviating and reapplied directly to the skin.

- Lavender Oil- Antifungal properties of this oil is effective for such conditions as, ringworm, jock itch, athletes foot also diminish the stinging of bug bites. This oil provides antibiotic, antioxidant and antiseptic properties that soothes and relaxes itchy skin disorders. Can be used or applied to your skin as needed after being mixed with a carrier oil.

- *Rose Geranium -Is an antifungal and antibacterial oil, used mostly to alleviate itching and dry skin. This oil can be mixed with Lavender and Chamomile oil for added benefits.*

   Remember what I mention earlier in chapters 2 and 3 how inflammation causes many illness and disorders well it effects the skin in this way also.

   There are many others oils that you can use, but these listed above counteract just about all skin disorders you could think, that effect the skin.

   I have found out of all the above mentioned oils, my use and results with tea tree oil to be one of the best ESO for treating skin disorders, because of it antibacterial properties to destroys many forms of outer.

This system as stated earlier in the book consist of 206 bones and is very essential to the overall functioning of our bodies, there are many aliments that attack our bones and I have found essential oils(ESO's) to be very beneficial in reducing pain and inflammation.

One of the most common diseases of the bones is Arthritis, there are many forms of it that cause debilitating pain and the inability to function.

Some ESO's I have used and received benefits from are listed below, there are many others such as lemongrass, lavender, ginger, clove bergamot, Frankincense and Myrrh all of these are great oils. Research and find out which of these oils work best for you.

- *Thyme - Rosemary - Sage - Theses oils are essential in reducing bone breakdown that leads to osteoporosis, which may occur as we age. There are also other forms of arthritis that effect bone health. Osteoarthritis, rheumatoid arthritis, childhood arthritis, Gout and Fibromyalgia. Massaging the area of the body where the bone pain is felt, will relieve the pain and decrease or diminish bone calcification. Use these oils separately with a carrier oil and often per day as needed at least 3-4 times and if used regularly for several weeks your joint will improve or diminish completely. When desired results are achieved continue daily use once a day to maintain wellness.*

- *Black Cumin Oil(aka) Black seed oil-This oil can be used directly out of the bottle. Rubbing it into the aching joint at least 2 - 3 times a day for several weeks will aid in reducing inflammation and swelling. Continue regiment as needed to maintain joint health. I suggest at least once a day.*

- *Remember your omegas 3, 6, and 9's along with Calcium, magnesium and vitamin 03 taken daily contributes to healthy bone health, especially as we age we lose a lot of these minerals from our bones, which causes them to become brittle and we can develop low bone density.*

- *Change of diet is very essential in obtaining bone health. Four to five servings of fruits, vegetables and whole grains are part of a healthy diet and contribute to healthy bones, decreases inflammation and can naturally help control your weight. Maintaining a healthy weight relieves stress on your joints, also decreasing your excess body fat by exercising at least 3 times a week or more, helps you to create a daily workout routine that lowers blood pressure, increase cardiac blood flow and gives you that all over good feeling of energy.*

I was diagnosed 5 years ago with osteoarthritis of both knees stage 0 mild but the change in my ambulation and mobility as well as pain was real. My physician said to me, you really have nothing to worry about at this time, there's no need for any treatment or none that can be done at this time. I started researching preventive care measures to assist and heed any further bone and cartilage breakdown to my knees. I found 2 oils that were well represented. Rosemary oil and Lemongrass oil. I mixed them separately to see which one would work best with a carrier oil. I used them on a trial basis for 7-10 days each. I obtained the best results with lemongrass and use it now daily 3-4 times a day, I massage it into my knees and my pain decrease to a minimum within 3 days and to none after 7- 10 days of usage. I've been able to resume light cardia and walking 3-5 times a week. I have been really pleased with the changes in my mobility ambulation and pain relief. I can't state enough to check with your physician before using or adding any new treatment to your medication regiment, because some ESO's can produce side effects that you may not be aware of that can cause contraindication to medication.

Chapter 11

The Skeletal System and Essential Oils

Essential oils can provide healthy skeletal support to our bones, joints, tendons and ligaments. A healthy skeletal support can include the use of essential oils and supplements to aid in maintaining healthy bones and joints.

The skeletal system is responsible for helping you maintain your mobility and joint function.

Listed are ESO that support in the healing of injuries to the bones. There are many oils that work in bone healing, but I want to inform you of the oils that work the best in bone healing.

Cypress Oil

Fir- needle oil,

Lemongrass oil

wintergreen oil

Best results occur when these oils are used with a carrier oil and massaged into the affected area 3-5 times daily, until desired results.

Herbs and supplements that aid bone health

Cassia- (Fabaceae) A plant herb also known as legumes family which consist of peas, beans all types such as chickpeas, soybeans, lentils, peanuts this plant herb is used for healing sprains, sore joints, fractures or broken bones.

Supplements that aid bone health are Calcium, Vitamin D and protein are important supplements to take every day to maintain healthy bones and aid in the healing of broken bones.

Turmeric has been effective in the and reduction of inflammation in the body it also has shown positive results for the bone healing and protection from disorders and formation of new bones.

Listed are some disease that can contribute to bone loss.

Autoimmune disorders, medical procedures, spinal cord injuries, depression, gastrointestinal disorders, eating disorders, endocrine and hormonal disorders blood bone marrow disorders and hematologic/ blood disorders.

Cinnamon oil Spice oil used as a massage oil when mixed with a carrier and massaged into the knees daily or 1-3 times a week helps to reduce bone breakdown and also help prevent Osteoporotic which means porous having spaces or holes in between the bones which causes fluid to pass through and causes osteoporotic arthritis.

Inflammation Juice Recipe; This will decrease inflammation within your entire body by 90% Blend together these ingredients in a juicer or blender. Purchase organic ingredients when possible.

1 granny smith apple

1 small cucumber

½ of a whole pineapple

1 cup spinach

1 peeled lemon

Juice all ingredients add ice and enjoy.

Drinking this juice daily for at least 21 days will reduce inflammation in your body, for routine maintenance consume at least once a week,

Chapter 12

The Muscular System and Essential oils.

The muscular system is a very powerful system it consists of 700 muscle throughout our bodies Essential oils (ESO's) is effective in relieving sore muscles, tension, pain and swelling. There are many oils on the market but I've found these to work best for me.

Frankincense Oil- (Boswellia Cartorii) This oil is considered the king of oils and is one of the most potent and medicinally useful ESO's on the planet. Its main benefit is boosting the immune system by stimulating your system to become active and into fight mode to kill any harmful germs and bacteria, which try to invade our bodies. This oil is mention in the bible mare than 54 time and used often by the physicians of this time. This oil can be used in creams lotions and salves by mixing

- 5-10 drops in your favorite ointment and messaging your body daily or as you prefer.

   I mix 10 drops with almond oil into a Rolette and carry with me daily, you may also use in a diffuser by adding 2-4 drops with water into a diffuser and allow it to diffuse into the air.

- Clary Sage Oil- Alleviates muscle tension and spasms while promoting relaxation.

- Ginger Oil- Provides a warming effect on sore muscles, which helps relieve pain.

- Black pepper Oil- alleviates pain by warming up the body.

- Cloves Oil- Treats painful sore muscles, also has a warming effect on them.

- Sandalwood Oil-Alleviates muscles spasms, tension and inflammation.

- Lavender Oil - Calms and relaxes sore muscles and also relieves pain and inflammation.

- Yarrow Oil- Is used to reduce pain and inflammation.

- Rosemary Oil Is noted for its ability to ease pain and inflammation.

- Eucalyptus Oils - provides a cooling effect to muscle pain and inflammation.

- *Peppermint Oil - contains menthol, which has a cooling effect on sore achy muscles. It also has analgesic antispasmodic and anti- inflammatory properties.*

- *Marjoram Oil - Relaxes muscles spasm and tension. It also eases pain and inflammation.*

- *Lemongrass Oil - Is one of the best oils for muscle pain and inflammation*

- *Ylang Yang Oil - Promotes relaxation and kills bacteria to open wounds when applied to the skin with a carrier oil, it also lower blood pressure.*

Remember the best natural remedy for muscles is Epsom salts with ½ cup of baking soda added to your bath water allow your body to soak for 15- 20 minutes will relieve achy muscles and joints.

These are some of the oils I have used as well as my family members and can speak on their benefits and effectiveness.

Chapter 13

Lymphatic System and Essential Oils

The lymphatic system is a very important and complex system, because it cleanses away metabolic waste produced by cells, tissues and organs. It also rids the body waste we accumulate in our bodies daily. Through research, I've discovered the best way to get rid your body of toxins is with using a dry brush, you can purchase a shower brush or a small hand held brush at any bath and beauty supply store, Walmart, Ross and many department stores that carry bath supplies, these usually cost between 5- 10 dollars, do invest in a sturdy brush for optimal benefits.

I usually brush my skin prior to taking a bath or shower, it allows your pores to open and stimulates the skin as well. Remember to always brush in an upward motion towards your heart and starting with your foot moving up lower legs, thigh, arm, chest, neck using short strokes toward the heart. I found it best to do one entire side of my body at a time and do the same process for the opposite side, this usually take me about 10 to 15 minutes to complete my entire body, I found a warm to tepid hot shower with a cool water rinse to allow your pores to close works best. Best if done at least 3 times a week, but you can also do daily if you prefer.

Some of the essential oils best used for lymph drainage are. Which also aids the body healing process of the included acute and chronic illnesses listed.

- *Peppermint oil-allergies, asthma, Bell's Palsy, chronic fatigue, hypothyroidism, morning sickness, joint pain, fainting, poor concentration and tension headaches*

- *Oregano oil- athlete's foot, boils, bronchitis, ringworm, strep throat, gangrene, planter warts and pancreatitis*

- *Orange oil - Anxiety, cold, detox, heartburn, insomnia, stress, sadness, fear and nausea*

- *Ginger root oil- Angina, constipation, gas, indigestion, vertigo motion sickness and scurvy*

- *Rosemary oil-Cancer, depression, respiratory infections, fatigue, hair loss, liver conditions, jaundice, memory and emotion balance*

- *Clove oil- Blood clots, cataracts abscess, chicken pox, Lyme disease, smoking, addiction, toothache, thrush, herpes, and gingivitis it can also destroy mold*

Remember to dilute these oils with a carrier oil before messaging it onto your skin, to avoid an allergic reaction. I recommend adding 1-2 drops to olive or coconut oil and massage each area of your body prior to massaging and brushing your skin. You can also dry brush and massage with these oils after your shower or bath_ I recommend adding 1-3 drops of oil of your choice to bath water, but use only, combination use can cause an allergic reaction, especially if you have sensitive skin, you can experiment with using these oils until you find the one you like and works best for your body I found peppermint works best for my skin, since I have dry skin now, due to menopause and /love the smell of it on my skin.

You can also do a foot detox that helps rid the body of toxins, check out Amazon for a sonic foot detoxing machine they cost between 30- 100 dollars depending on the brands.

I use the Better home company brand for the last several years and found it to be very beneficial to my overall health and wellbeing. Follow the institutions that come with it, you'll find it worth the investment.

Chapter 14

The Circulatory system and essential oils

The use of essential oils with the circulatory system is to improve the blood flow in the body. There are many oils that can be used but, I've found these oils to be recommended as the best ones to use.

- Cypress oil
- Coriander oil
- Eucalyptus oil
- Black pepper oil
- Ginger Oil
- Cumin oil
- Wintergreen oil
- Lavender oil
- Neroli oil
- Juniper oil
- Rosemary oil

Remember to use a good quality (EO) and make sure it's organic and a brand that you trust. Here's a recipe you can use if you suffer with circulatory issues, consult your physician before using, because some diseases and chronic illness may deter your health. Recipe I use:

- 2-5 drops of black pepper essential oil
- 2-5 drops of rosemary essential oil

I mix these 2 oils together with 30 ml of a carrier oil and massage onto my skin after my bath or shower or you can also add just add 3-5 drops of one or both to your bath and soak for 15-20 minutes.

I recommend using only 1 of the essentials oil listed above due to possible allergic reactions that could occur. Try each oil for 7 days this way you'll able to learn which one benefits you best for your body, so you'll be able to minimize and know if it causes any allergic reaction to your body, such as coughing, wheezing, itching rash and other allergens and with the process of elimination you'll find out which oil works best for you. If you purchase an organic brand you should be fine.

Chapter 15

The Nervous System and essential oils

Essential oils are a great source for supporting the nervous system, due to their direct link to the limbic lobe of the brain, which is the emotional control center this area of the brain deals with and controls our emotion, depression, anxiety, fear anger, joy and varying emotions that we deal with on a daily basis including stress triggers.

Remember in the body systems I explained about the Central nervous function as well as the Peripheral nervous system.

These systems also support both parasympathetic and sympathetic nervous systems, Parasympathetic relates to the part of the automatic nervous system that counter balances the sympathetic nerves, which consist of the nerves arising from the brain and lower end of the spinal cord and supplying the internal organs, blood vessels and glands.

Essential oils for this system are better used in a diffuser you can add 3-5 drops to water that has been added as directed to your home diffuser. The oils are very relaxing and soothing to the entire body.

(ESO) I use as well as recommend:

- *Lavender oil*
- *Valerian root oil*
- *Ylang-ylang*
- *Patchouli*
- *Frankincense*

There are many other oils that you can use also, I recommend these in which I have used with good result.

You may also try Valerian root herbal capsules or tablets take as directed. I've found it to be a great relaxer. I usually take one capsule at bedtime and am able to sleep well and awaken refreshed in the morning. I only take if I've had stressful day. Be sure to check with your physician especially if you're on prescription medications.

Try them one at time for 7 days, remember to mix the ESO with a carrier oil if applying to the skin. The best pulse pressure points to apply ESO are in the bend of the elbows, in the center of your throat, behind your ears, left side of chest below the heart, wrist, ankles and bottom of your feet. You will need to apply ESO for several times throughout the day for best results. Repeat the process with each oil to find out which one offers you the best benefits.

Remember the nervous system is one of the most delicate and essentials systems of the body it's made up of 7 trillion nerve cells its similar to driving on the highway. The nervous system communicates brain which the senses carries your thought and actions throughout your body from the tip of your toes to the top your head. It's make it possible for your sense to work, for your brain to think, your limbs to move, and for all your various organs to do their jobs without your conscious input.

ESO can help you keep you establish, maintain, and optimize basic health habits to keep your nervous system healthy. Balance the sympathetic and parasympathetic branches of your nervous system. Possibly reduce the symptoms of neurodegenerative disease like Alzheimer's, dementia and neuropathy.

ESO are good for aiding people that suffer with mental health issues, depression, anxiety, bipolar schizophrenia and many others. Depression and anxiety are the most prevalent mental illness worldwide. Of over 4.4% and 3.6%, respectively.

Remember to get plenty of sleep, the nervous system communicates better when the body is well rested.

I added some other herbs that can be very beneficial in aiding calm to the nervous system.

- *Holy Basil*
- *Chamomile*
- *Lemon Balm*
- *Passion Flower*
- *Skull Cap*
- *Gotu Kola*
- *Kava Kava*
- *Bacopa*
- *Motherwort*
- *Ashwagandha*

These herbs can be purchase in capsules, tablet and tea form, before taking in pill form make sure to check with your physician, if taking prescription medication and only take as your physician directs or as directed on manufacturer bottle before adding to your medication regimen.

You can also use these oils in a diffuser, its best to use at night in your bedroom while you sleep, it causes the body to be in a relaxed state and awake refreshed. I have several diffusers in my home and use them throughout the day, it provides with a calm physical, mental and spiritual relaxation throughout the day.

Chapter 16

The Respiratory System and essential Oils

The respiratory tract has a thin, moist lining called the mucus membrane, which can become inflamed as a result of infection or allergic reactions. Swelling of the affected membrane narrows the nasal passages and makes breathing more difficult. Sometimes secondary infections such as, sinusitis, bronchitis, flu, and the common cold may also develop. Certain essential oils will help to reduce inflammation and loosen mucus, others have strong antiseptic properties that help fight infection.

Here are some that have been used favorably, with good results.

- Eucalyptus is one of the best oils used for respiratory health
- Rosemary promotes healthy respiratory function especially congestion caused by a cold or the flu. It's also beneficial for improving sleep, reducing anxiety and relieving minor pain and inflammation, especially relating to stressed out and tense muscles.
- Peppermint oil promotes antiseptic and anti-spasmodic, effective in reducing mucus, and relieving coughs, throat infections, asthma and bronchitis, flu, colds, and sinusitis. Use in bath by adding 5-7 drops in your water and relaxing for 15-20 minutes.
- White Fir soothes muscles and increases poor circulation inhibits bronchial infections and reduces asthma and coughing
- Lemon mix with carrier oil and massage onto skin around the throat area several times throughout the day, it has a calming effect and fights bacteria.
- Frankincense is valued for its immune strengthening capabilities and beneficial effects on the respiratory system. It is an antiseptic and anti-inflammatory to the lung, when used in a diffuser or adding a few drops into hot water and covering your head with a towel and inhaling it can reduce nasal inflammation of the respiratory tract, relieving cough, mucus, asthma, bronchitis

These oils can be mixed with a carrier oil and rubbed onto the skin several times a day. Used in a diffuser 3-5 drops mixed with water and diffused in your home throughout the day

Inhaled adding 5-8 drops in a glass bowel half filled with hot water in a glass and using a towel to cover your head while placing your face over the bowel to and inhale for 10 -20 minutes its beneficial in opening up the lungs and riding them of mucus while relieving the sinus passages of inflammation and swelling, making breathing easier.

There are many other ESO that are beneficial, but these are the ones I and my family have used with great results.

So remember the 7-day rule use one ESO at a time for 7 days, before trying another one and monitoring the effects.

Chapter 17

The Reproductive System and Essential Oils

The reproductive system deals with the anatomy of the female body. I will discuss ESO that assist in the healing of our bodies. Many women face challenges that concerns their daily health as well, such as, menstrual cramps, endometriosis, bloating as well as pregnancy and fertility concerns.

There are many ESO you can use, but I would like to give you a few of the oils mostly used today.

- *Geranium oil: known to be beneficial in relieving menstrual cramps.*

- *Cary Sage oil: known and used for menopausal relief when using this particular oil, be sure you are not pregnant the use of it can be toxic to you due to your hormonal changes in your body while pregnant.*

- *Chamomile oil: Known as a very calming oil and is used, for abdominal pain, bloating and contraction, this oil works better in cream form you can add 5-10 drops to a carrier oil and massaged into the abdomen as needed for relief and comfort can also use in a diffuser.*

- *Cypress oil: Know and used mostly for varicose vein, hemorrhoids and strengthening the blood vessels in the body and improving circulation, especially during pregnancy.*

- *Lavender oil: Known to be a relaxing and good stress reliever during pregnancy, used in a diffuser and relax.*

- *Peppermint oil: it has been known to aid in relieving headaches and migraines which have been linked to endometriosis, which is associated with infertility.*

- *Orange and Lemon oils: Orange oil has been known to lessen anxiety in women that are in labor, Lemon oil: Is best known to alleviate nauseous stomach, during pregnancy.*

- *Sandalwood oil: Know to benefits men's testosterone levels and women's libido when used as a cream or diffused in a room diffuser prior to sexual activity, when trying to conceive.*

These oil can be used with a carrier oil by adding 4-8 drops in organic oil of your choice and use as needed, or you may want to purchase these oils in cream form and massage your body as directed per instructions.

Remember to check with your gynecologist if pregnant, before using any ESO. It's very important to protect your unborn child as well as yourself.

Chapter 18

The Immune System and Essential Oils

Your lifestyle can affect how well your immune system can protect you from germs, virus, and chronic illness. Replacing bad habits with good ones is a great way to start. Such as changing your diet, making it healthier, exercising, getting enough sleep at least 8 hours, finding ways to distress by doing meditations, and taking out 1 hour a day for just you. I call that ME time, by going to a quiet place in your home and Jet everyone in your household know that you don't wish to be disturb until that hour is up. Taking a vitamin C tablets daily 500 to 1000 mg daily helps to build the immune system against germ especially in the fall and winter months. ESO that benefit the immune system.

- *Tea Tree oil: best known for its immune system support and microbial properties and its ability to stimulate the immune system, which helps fight off infection and disease. It is an oil that can be used daily.*

- *Eucalyptus oil: Know and used as a decongestant that can help clear up respiratory ailments, such as, the cold and flu, also fights the bacteria that causes infections, such as, step, tuberculosis, and MRSA.*

- *Oregano oil: Known for its powerful healing properties its antibacterial, antiviral and has immune promoting properties. These properties also make oregano great for fighting infection, an important part of maintaining a healthy immune system.*

- *Lemon oil: Known for its use as a body detoxifier, because of its abundance of vitamins and minerals. It contains the properties of the fruit itself Lemon can also be used to improve mood, and sharpen focus.*

- *Lavender oil: known for its benefit and ability to relieve stress, which is one of the biggest factors in promoting immune system health. Lavender is filled with antioxidants that remove free radicals from our system which are often associated with cell damage, illness, and aging.*

Essential Oil Blend for Immune support. Immunity blend you can use.4 drops of lavender. 2 drops of eucalyptus and 1 drop of tea tree oil this mixture can be diffused in a room diffuser or mixed with a carrier oil and applied daily as needed.

Chapter 19

Endocrine System

Essentials oils used to aid and support the healthy functioning of the endocrine system varies.

- Rosemary Oil
- Clary Sage Oil
- Lemongrass Oil
- Rose Oil
- Melissa Oil
- Fennel Oil

The first 3 oils mentioned are my favorite oils to use in a diffuser or 2--5 drops added to a carrier oil of your choice and massaged into the skin area of choice inner arms, wrist abdomen, thighs or lower legs.

There are many diseases that effects the endocrine system, but I've found Diabetes, to be the most Chronic disease of the endocrine system that effects millions of people.

Diabetes is known to effects the pancreas through its over production of sugar spilling into the blood stream which can cause hyper which is high blood sugar levels in the body or hypo which is low blood sugar that are control with the use of insulin or diabetic oral medications.

The functioning of the pancreas is essential to the functioning of the adrenal glands, which are located on top of the kidneys. The adrenal glands produce many important hormones, including cortisol, aldosterone and adrenaline. The adrenal hormone helps regulate several bodily functions including metabolism, blood pressure and your body response to stress.

Diabetes contributes to poor blood flow circulation of the upper and lower extremities, slow healing of wounds, blurred eyesight that can lead to deterioration of vision, which can contribute to blindness, there are so many acute and chronic ailments and diseases of the endocrine system that you may want to check them out on this website **endocrine web. com** for more information especially if you are dealing with an illness or diseases related to the endocrine system.

Many children suffer wit diabetes and chronic ailments as well as diseases of the endocrine system.

Make sure to check with your child's pediatrician before using any essential oils, due to the toxic effects it could cause to their body.

The top 11 organic essential oil companies I recommend and have used are listed.

- Plant Therapy
- Doterra
- Rocky Mountain Oils,
- Young Living
- Arts Naturals
- Eden Garden
- Revive
- Vitruvi
- Aesthetics Naturals,
- Calily
- Plant Guru

The Endocrine system is a very complex system so be careful when using ESO consulting with your Physician is strongly advised before using.

- Young Living
- Arts Naturals
- Eden Garden
- Revive
- Vitruvi
- Aesthetics Naturals,
- Calily
- Plant Guru

The Endocrine system is a very complex system so be careful when using ESO consulting with your Physician is strongly advised before using.

Chapter 20

The Digestive System and Essential Oils

The digestive system and oils that aid in this systems wellbeing, your digestive system plays an important role in breaking down of food and absorbing nutrients into the blood stream, also remember that inflammation within your body cause stomach ailments, leaky gut stomach gastrointestinal symptoms, such as, stomach problems, diarrhea, heartburn bloating abdominal pain, constipation_ nausea/vomiting, dysphagia and bowel incontinence. ESO used to aid these aliments.

- *Ginger oil: Stimulates the digestive system, which stimulates the digestive system, which increases gastric activity, thus helping to prevent and alleviate constipation.*

- *Green Mandarin oil: known best for easing the mind and producing sleep, which provides secondary digestive benefits.*

- *Digest Ease oil: Known for its healing properties, which is an oil you can purchase Doterra it's a combination of different combinations already blended together and ready for use to be mixed in a carrier oil and applied to the abdomen as needed for stomach discomfort or pain.*

- *Fennel oil: Known to aid in the relief of constipation, mix with a carrier oil and massage on your abdomen in order to enjoy the digestive benefits*

- *Cloves Bud oil: Know best for easing digestive upset, stomach aches, acid reflux it can also help relax your mind and your nerves, which in turn help soften stomach issues.*

These are just a few of the best known oils that help alleviate digestive aliments.

Chapter 21

Urinary System

The urinary system eliminates waste from the body it also is considered the body's drainage system for the eventual removal of urine. It is very important for us to drink at least 8 oz. of water daily to assist your body in staying hydrated.

One of the main diseases that can cause permanent kidney damage is chronic hypertension (aka) high blood pressure. Uncontrolled high blood pressure can lead to complete renal failure, which leads many people to hemodialysis or peritoneal dialysis. Both my parents lived with this disease and had to be dialyzed 3 times a week for the rest of their lives.

It's very important to take care of your kidneys and bladder because these two organs work coincide with other. Even with medication many people still have uncontrollable high blood pressure. I myself have suffer with this chronic illness since my late SO's and have been prescribed many different medications under my doctor's supervision to control this silent killer. That contributes also to strokes, chronic headaches, daily general fatigue, brain *fog*, aneurisms, blood clots and overall damage to the entire body.

I found hypertension to be a contributor to many illnesses we suffer with today and very hard to control even with medication, I found essential oil's usage for the urinary system, to be limited, to the use of teas herbs, and supplements, that assist in preventing urinary tract infections.

- Cranberry Tea
- Green Tea
- Chamomile Tea
- Mint tea
- Parsley Tea

These teas might be better for the immune system than antibiotics because they can help soothe the irritation and speed up the healing process.

They can also help you stay hydrated and staying hydrated is very important if you've got a UTI.

They contain anti - inflammatory and antiseptic properties which can cure itching and irritation, killing the bad bacteria from urine.

Herbal teas also help to strengthen your bladder creating a healthy environment.

Another tea I found to be very helpful is **Dandelion Tea** because of its anti-bacteria compound it may help to prevent urinary tract infections. You do need to be careful with this tea because it can cause an allergic reaction. Check with your physician before drinking this tea it may also interact negatively with medications. I pair it with one of the above listed teas and have had no issues, but remember what's good for one-person system may reacts differently with yours, so try one tea at a time for several days to assure you don't have an allergic reaction before paring with dandelion tea, since it is very potent tea.

There are essential oils that can be used aid in the prevention of UTI's, when used with a carrier oil and massaged into the right and left lower outer sides of the back, you can use daily or 2-3 times a week.

- Lemongrass Oil
- Oregano Oil
- Clove Oil
- Cinnamon Oil
- Tea Tree Oil
- Thyme Oil
- Lavender Oil
- Eucalyptus Oil is considered the universal oil it's a good option to use when a person is unsure which type of bacteria is causing the infection.

There are many others, but I've found these to work best remember to try one oil at a time this will help you find the one that works best for you and don't forget to check with your physician before using especially if you are taking medications.

These oils can also be used in a diffuser 2-5 drops added to purified water not tap water unless you have a water filter on your faucet that help remove contaminates from your water.

Chapter 22

DIY (Do It Yourself)

The following dilution guidelines are the recommended aromatherapy standards: There are 2 tablespoons in 1 ounce.

The chart attached is for both tablespoons and ounces.

Included is a chart you can use ESO for adults, infants and children.

OUNCES

Infants & Children:

0.5% = 3 drops of EOS per ounce of carrier oil

1% = 6 drops of EOS per ounce of carrier oil

Adults

2% = 12 drops of ESO per ounce of carrier oil

3% = 18 drops of ESO per ounce of carrier oil

5% = 30 drops of EOS per ounce of carrier oil

105 = 60 drops of ESO per ounce of carrier oil

TABLESPOONS

Infants & Children

0.5% = 1.5 of ESO per tablespoon of carrier oil

1% = 3% of ESO per tablespoon of carrier oil

Adults

2% = 6 drops of ESO per tablespoon of carrier oil

3% = 9 drops of ESO per tablespoon of carrier oil

5% =15 drop of ESO per tablespoon of carrier oil

10% = 30 drops of ESO per tablespoon of carrier oil

Chapter 23

Herbs and Supplements that promote Optimal Health and Well-Being

Introduction: Composed is a detailed list of herbs and vitamins supplements that I've research and used for their potential benefits, as they relate to the healing of certain illness and disease of the body.

These herbs can be taken with your routine medications. You should check with your physician and research for any contraindications that can occur such as allergies.

1. *Vitamins and supplements that aid High blood pressure aka (HTN) Potassium 300 mg per day*

   Garlic supplement 500mg twice a day or 100 mg once a day use the odorless cold process if you can find it.

   Omega 3 fatty fish oil500 to 1000 mg per day or an organic Co Q10 supplement once daily.

   Multivitamin one per day

   Magnesium Chelate 250mg twice a day

2. *Inflammation of the joints: Dr. Axe Multi Collagen Protein supplement comes in powder and capsule form is one of the best products I have taken that has aided my joint health improvement by 90%*

   Vitamin D3 is good for the bones take as directed daily

   Vitamin K+2 take as directed usually daily

   Glucosamine plus Chondroitin take daily as directed per package directions

3. *Gastrointestinal: GI ailments such as Cohn's disease, Ulcerative colitis, Diverticulitis and others:*

   Vitamin D 600 units per day

   Iron 1 tablet per day

Folic acid one tablet per day

Vitamins A, E and K one tablet per day

Zinc one tablet a day

These vitamins are considered fat soluble vitamins and minerals that aid in vitamin deficiencies that can occur to the colon due to poor diet and food nutrition. They support stabilization of your digestive system.

4. *Memory Loss long and Short term:*

   Ginkgo Biloba: improves memory concentration take one tablet or capsule as directed

   DMAE: Improves mood, alertness and focus Take as tablet or capsule as directed Acetyl -L Carnite: A Brain antioxidant which helps prevent brain and cell deterioration, a potent fat burner

   Vinopocetine: a powerful memory enhancer

   Improves cognitive performance

   Provides strong effects to cerebral circulation and blood flow to the brain. TAKE THESE SUPPLEMENTS AS DIRECTED BY PHYSICAN OR MANUFACTURER

5. *Peripheral Neuropathy: Wheatgrass is a great herb that can be taken in powder, liquid or pill form, aids in alleviating tingling sensations of the nerves.*

6. *Black Seed Oil is highly recommended supplement that is known as the cure all supplement of over 100 aliments, illness and diseases of the body.*

Remember that illness and diseases arise from a buildup of inflammation in the body especially GI and digestive aliments and our heritage as well as our family history play a big part in our health issues.

Black Seed oil will aid in decreasing inflammation in your body which causes the body to become healthy and whole along with diet changes and daily aerobic exercise can aid you in living a healthy and fulfilled life

Take 1 teaspoon of Black seed oil twice a day with honey due to the taste of the oil it is pungent. You can also take 1 teaspoon as a tea in warm water in the morning and at bedtime.

Thank You for purchasing my book I pray it benefits your health as it has benefited my family and myself. True health begins with you, be you own physician and heal yourself.

Printed in the United States
by Baker & Taylor Publisher Services